Phases

Of

Nunit

Phases Of Nunit

By: Bryona L. Lawrence

Copyright 2021 Bryona L. Lawrence

Bryona L. Lawrence on KDP

Atlanta, Ga

ISBN: #9781736120217

Introduction

Hello all, my name is Bryona Lawrence, I'm from Flint, MI. I was raised in a large family where there were more girls than boys.

I wrote this book mainly to vent my feelings, but I also realized this could possibly help someone. In my few years here on earth, I have been through a lot. I am grateful for the strength that has kept me going.

I have learned to appreciate what I have, and to be thankful. I put this book together not for sympathy, but to help someone who can relate to me.

I am thankful to those who support me, and all of the life lessons that has inspired this collection of poetry. As an expression of my gratitude, I would like to leave you with these tokens. I've learned that people come, people go but that is okay. Having everything figured out comes with time. Lastly, Reader, you should know that I accept you for who you are, and I wish you the best of luck and prosperity. Enjoy.

Table Of Contents

I Was Angry Once...

Brought to me from the stars, he was blessed with grace. I was down on my knees, yelling I need space. But what I really needed, was just to see my father's face. A broken-hearted young girl, trying to fill in that space.

In this world full of confusion, my young heart roared with rage, banging heavily against my chest, like an old 808 bass. Bottling up my anger, as I prayed for better days. Daddy you should have stuck around, I wished you would have stayed.

Daddy I have searched for your love, and I am so ashamed. Looking back at my past, I have done some dishonorable things. I have done the unthinkable, thinking it would bring me change. Instead, I end-up feeling empty, with a rotation of men.

Daddy I wish you were here with me, to help me avoid these sins, because these men do not love me, they just want my gem.

Maybe we can build one day, but for now I think I am ok. Because if you really loved me, like a father, you would have just stayed. Even with all the praying I did, you still managed to walk away. But you should know by now, that turning your back on me, was your very first mistake.

Fill My Cup...

I need a King, but he will need to have patience, because my mind can run off into the deep end at times, it causes sticky situations.

Listening to me rant, even when I'm yellin, because he is aware, there's some hell within heaven.

I need him to be kind, as he makes love to my spirit. Encourage me when I want to give up, even when he doesn't wanna hear it.

Be my peace, love, and light, with no unresolved issues. The shoulder I can cry on, no need for a tissue.

Understand these phases of me, don't see them as flaws. Protect me from this world full of chaos, where we can conquer it all.

I refuse to accept less, for I hold the throne. But until I heal myself within, I'm better off alone.

Use Your Voice

If this road ends here, who will stand with me? Will you help fight for our *freedom*, so we can live in *peace*?

Will you fight for my rights in private, like you do in front of me? All we ask for is *love, peace*, and *equality*.

The war has never ended, and the fight has never stopped. America building a perception of us, labeling *Black* people as things we are not.

Wanting us to be silent, while you water the soils with our blood. All we do is ask for *respect*, and to you that is asking for too much.

You want us to be a slave still, in *Great America*. Taking what is ours, well how is that fair to us?

You thought we would be *fearful*, but we are ready for war. Just like the police system, we shoot, kill, and destroy.

As long as we have a tongue, you will hear what we have to say. We have our *Ancestors* on our side, so we aren't easily swayed.

We shoot back in this generation; this isn't back in the day. We are awakening to our true *purpose*, so *you should* be afraid.

Realization

The sun went down today, and the darkness began to fill my room, I ran my daily bath to calm my mind, as the demons continued to feed off of my wounds,

I began washing my hair, detangling strand by strand, chanting positive mantras, as my happiness floats away with the wind,

I realized that I could be so peaceful, if I just loved myself within, but I am too busy chasing happiness, which leaves me hurt, empty, and broken,

I don't want to be deemed as damaged, but sometimes it's how I feel, I don't want to be deemed as unstable; but these wounds seem like they may never heal,

I tend to carry my heart on my sleeve, while my feelings hang outside of my chest, but now that I've learned how to protect them, maybe that will relieve some of my stress?

Trying To Let It Go

I can't explain why I feel this way, I just can't express how I feel, tears run down my face as I write, these emotions seem so unreal,

I am just a girl who cries alone, and of course, I barely sleep, I am just a girl who holds onto hope, who tries to stay away from confusion, I prefer peace,

Putting smiles on the faces of others, but I seem to forget about myself, giving love to all the wrong people, who only care about my wealth,

You would think I'd have it figured out, by the way I fix my crown, you would think I'd be outspoken, by the words I'm bold enough to write down,

But, inside I still feel broken, I'm sorry, I must confess this now, I've been thinking about overdosing, just taking the simple way out,

It's a shame, because I'm so great, surely, I should wanna live, but even with the good, my mind still avoids the positive.

Friends

I'm a loyal person, especially if I call you friend, there's not many who hold that title, in fact, I can count them on one hand,

There's a lot of people who try to surround me, but they're not even right within, there's too many people who try to doubt me, but they ain't even got no wins,

Stop throwin' that word around loosely, I promise you people are whack, stop throwin that word around loosely, that's wasted energy you can't get back,

Words can be used as curses, now you're in the palm of their hand, be aware of who you keep company, I said, not everyone is your friend.

Stubborn

Stubborn I am, stubborn I may be, a quality I have, and a simple part of me,

I want to be perfect, so I must not rush, I'm here to give my best, no harm, and no fuss,

Mystical mind I have, such a brilliant one, I know, it's a compliment to me, so I'll never let it go,

Tryna keep an open mind, while fighting the urge to give up, putting faith and guidance into my Ancestors, they hold the last of my trust,

My stubbornness pushed that dark halo, right from above my head, I felt like a walking corpse, Yes, I was somewhat dead,

My brain produced thoughts of happiness, but my spirit was numb, but because of my stubbornness, I was able to stay strong,

I Want More For You

Let 'em be free in these dead ass streets,

Where he wanna be,

Let em go screw all these girls unprotected,

Making babies out of misery,

He wants to be the top player,

Even though he is almost 53,

Breaking women down into pieces,

Because he is hurt and angry,

Talkin' 'bout breaking generational curses,

But he still hasn't changed a thing,

He likes to change his women like purses,

He doesn't know he's a king,

But you have done your part,

Let em find his own dreams,

No use in sitting around,

When he doesn't feel a thing.

The Antidote

Why you do this to me?

You make me feel so calm that I end up falling into the wrong hands,

You make me forget my sorrows, the lessons that I have learned within,

Feeling like a forever spinning hurricane, but when I inhale you, I become balanced,

Boosting my confidence, you make me feel less damaged,

I told myself I would not buy you today, but we both knew I lied,

I am no good at budgeting, but for you, money is put to the side,

You have got a hold on me; you may have become my best friend,

When I inhale you, I feel less stressed, feeling like I can breathe again,

You are the melody to my tunes, so, I had to spark you up my friend,

Slowly becoming part of my DNA, as I take a puff, strand by strand.

Billion- Dollar Vibes

No one is playing hard to get, I am hard to get.

If I was so foolish to give all my jewels away, what else would I have left?

I am not the one for playing games, because I just don't have the time.

I am more up for building and uplifting; I call it billion-dollar vibes.

Dancing In Victory

My spirit dances in the world's open wounds, I've been tryin' to break generational curses and patterns,

Looking to the sky, as I jump and scream for clarity, hoping to get rid of some of this lifetime baggage,

I assume some people look up to me, so lately I've been tryna break bad habits,

And even with the critics in society's cruel world, I still somehow manage,

Manage to get up and smile, as I make my bed living lavish,

I figured it was a better choice to be happy, then to cry all day and be depressed,

I cannot afford to give you control over my emotions, or to treat me less than an empress,

I've been working hard on me, I won't allow you to backtrack my progress.

Just Breathe

I can be speechless at times, it scares me how much love
I carry,

It scares me to the point, that I sometimes have anxiety
attacks,

It scares me that my love might not ever be reciprocated,
or given back,

"There goes my anxiety again", I say, as I fight to catch
my breath,

I squeeze my right hand, with my face frowning up,
trying to control what happens next,

This is one of my bad days, the days I truly just wish to
rest,

I start breathing in and out, counting to twenty-five, to
relieve the pressure from my chest,

Spirit, you ask me not to love so hard, and to try and be
patient,

But why should I hide who I am? They should love me
for all of my phases.

Miracle

I had a dream about you, Miracle. I dreamt that my sister would give birth alone, and that she would be afraid. It is almost as if I felt her pain and sorrow, running through my very own veins.

Perhaps her reactions are based on the emotions, that we both refuse to display; you see, I love your mother, even though she may not feel that way.

My sister has always carried so much love for people, my honey just wanted the same; for someone to hold on to her and, tell her she will be safe.

If she feels this way Miracle, then we really are one of the same. All that time I had been judging her, I was really reflecting on me.

All this time, I've been using the wrong words to describe your mother; she's a force to be reckoned with, and has the heart of a lover.

It's 2020, and I'm just now figuring out what she was missing. She was missing you, Miracle. You are her peace and her hope. You are the very thing that will make her fall in love with herself again. You are the key to her heart, and what will keep her calm. You are her step into reality, into adulthood.

Even though your name is not Miracle, you are a Miracle to my sister. You even came out as a fighter early, three months to be exact. Once they showed me your picture, lightweight and all, you still looked like fat. You are my sisters' happiness; about the only thing she does not regret.

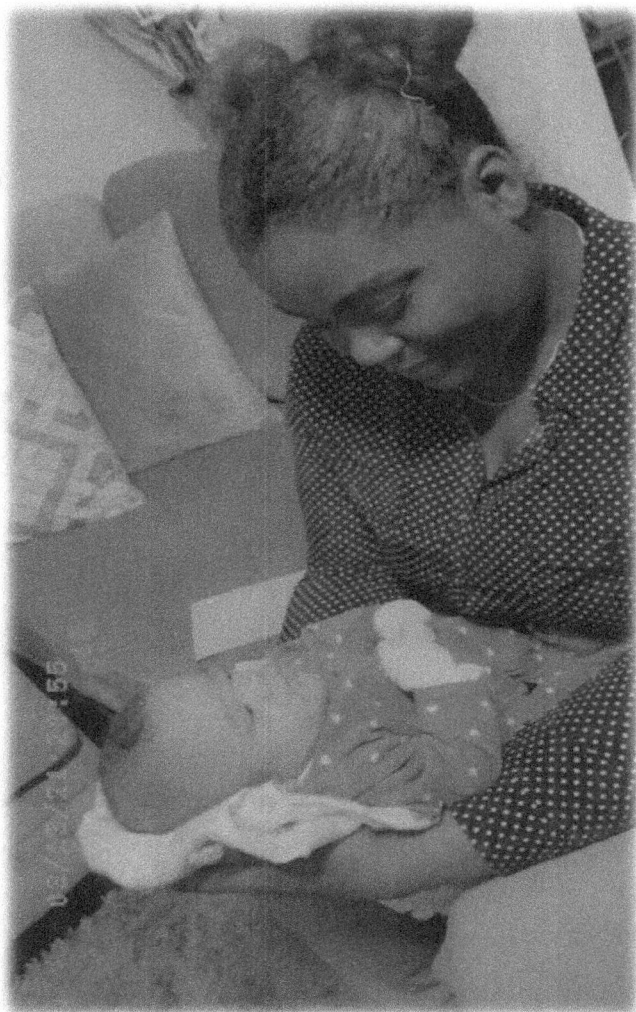

My Second Niece

New Arrival

It all started with a baby girl; a baby girl being had by my Baby Girl.

I can still remember when you used to sleep all day as a baby, whiny. I remember you breaking into the fridge. Now I sit holding your hand, as you are trying to catch your breath.

April 4th was the very first time I witnessed a live birth. Witnessing a live baby being pulled from below.

I was so confused, not knowing if I should be happy or downright afraid. Not knowing how being a young mother would affect you, sister.

But as soon as I looked into the eyes of my first niece, my worries disappeared; I could have sworn it was a dream.

She was just so beautiful; I knew that God had blessed our family. This would be our first step of possibly healing, creating a loving space.

We will help you to become a woman, as you humble us along the way. Helping the family to forget about ego, you are the light that will keep us sane.

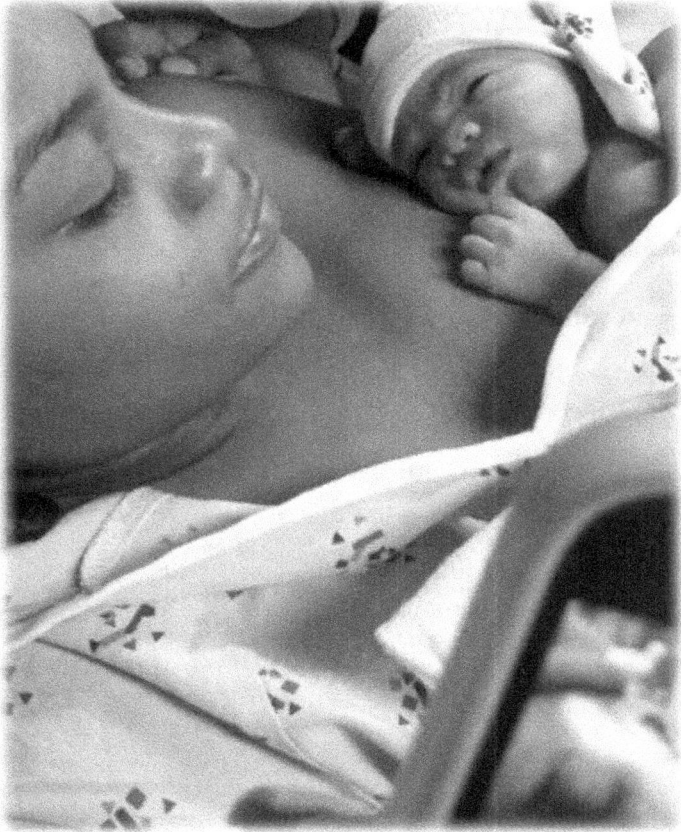

My First Niece

Dick Distractions

Walking down the sidewalk, trying to free my mind. The goal is to be grounded and steady,

Conflicts inside my heart, issues sitting on my spine. My pussy is hot and ready,

My phone buzzed, and I'm afraid to look down, because I will go against my own intuition,

I will be left in a bed, full of tears. This is one of my least intelligent decisions,

He is the type of man, I know I should avoid, because it interrupts my positive transition,

But in this moment, he's stroking me from behind, as I'm forced to take what he is givin',

Ending up on my knees, not coming up for air. Posing like I was going into meditation,

Even though I am sucking him, he is sucking me. I can feel my energy being taken,

This is not worth it at all, being left in your head, waking up at night sweating,

Give us the strength to walk away, and be smart and ignore these dick distractions.

Lies We Tell

You got what I need baby, I want your body all over me,
I can see how bad you want me, but would you be down
just to hold me?

Sometimes your girl gets lonely, and that's when you see
the hoe in me start wanting you to dig deep, lick, kiss,
and fuck on me,

I want a friend maybe a homie, I say as I am moanin',
using my pussy power, to cover up these emotions,

You said don't catch feelings, but I can't help it in the
moment; you shouldna kissed me like that, if you didn't
want nothin',

You see sometimes your girl gets lonely, and I may bust
it open, but he has to be of age, and eat this pussy like
his daily devotion,

You can't trust these niggas, closing my heart, just as fast
as it opened, sex won't fill the void, though that's what I
was hopin'.

I Cried When I Wrote This...

You really drove me crazy...

I was thinking about what you meant to me, and I have come to realize it was not love; it was misery.

Damn right you didn't deserve me. I know you're aware of how much you hurt me!

But I choose not to hold it against you, knowing me, I already had issues.

But it wasn't love, you were just ruthless with me. It was never love, it was just you mentally abusing me.

Using my mind to help keep your sanity. In fact, you'll never be considered a man to me.

Hurting me like you had something to prove to me, treating me like a peasant; I accepted it foolishly.

I am blessed your darkness didn't pass to me, because then I would be like you, living hatefully.

Dysfunctional...

Stuck in your own mind,

A place where no one knows,

Deep in your own tears, this is dysfunctional,

Hiding your pain, as you crack those smiles,

Choosing all the wrong paths,

You are stuck in denial,

You don't want counseling,

You'd rather hang out with friends,

Because then you can play forgetful,

Oh yes, the great game of pretend,

This is being dysfunctional,

What don't you comprehend?

This is being dysfunctional,

What don't you understand?

We've been lying to ourselves,

Saying we feel fine,

Meanwhile, your heart feels overwhelmed,

Holding yourself as you cry,

We search for love,

Instead of loving ourselves,

We would rather keep our minds in prison,

And endure the hell,

My darling this is dysfunctional,

I hope you get well,

I hope your heart heals from the damage,

But I guess only time will tell.

Communication...

My heart began beating, making the blood rush to my ears. My hands were shaking as I began typing, trying to form a sentence. I erased and retyped, over and over again. Feeling guilty of my actions, but the truth is I missed my friend.

I said that I hated you, but I was just disappointed. The time we have been apart, I was forced to deal with my emotions. I was forced to let go, and to heal myself from within. So, I typed "How are you?" and then I hit send.

I was at work, so anxious to see if you would reply. It made me self-reflect even more, because it was not just you, it was I. Even though everyone disagrees, you were still my prize. And no matter how hard I tried to forget, thoughts of you, weighed heavily on my mind.

But that perception is my fault, because I spoke of you as a villain. I supposed that is a common factor, in most hurt women. I wish I could take it all back, and change some of my decisions. The main decision would be, to keep people out of our business.

My Secret Love Desire

Every inch of your skin, I want to make love to. I want to caress your mind, fill it with joy, hope, and desire.

I want to suck your skin, like bees suck nectar from flowers. I want to just love you for you, and not the money you think gives you power.

Don't you feel our energy, my little secret love desire?

I can just imagine if we were together, but I suppose we will never know. Because I lack the confidence to fully open-up, and with those insecurities, we will never grow.

I stare at you sometimes, but I never approach. Maybe things are better off this way, because I still need to grow.

But, my secret love, I would love to have a family. Building an empire with you, although, I know I can be demanding.

Today you walked past, and I almost passed out. The letter was in my pocket, but my heart filled with doubts.

Panicking, I tried to head the opposite way, but as I began to turn, you decided to call my name. I stood still like death, not knowing what to say.

"What do you want?", I replied with sass. Then my eyes got big, when I saw what he had.

Patting my back pocket, thinking, "oh shit this is bad." I reached out to grab it, but then he tugged back. "Is this meant for me, because it says my name on the back?"

How Are You? Part 2

May I ask you a direct question, a simple one really?

How have you been doing, darling, how are you feeling?

You seem upset, and that energy is not appealin',

You seem so let down, but I am willing to listen,

I do not want to gossip, on whatever you tell me,

For I'm on a mission, to give you positive energy,

I just want to uplift you, ensure that you grow with me,

Ground yourself, darling, it is what you need,

You seem a little tired, I hope you can open-up to me,

You seem a little suicidal, and that really worries me,

You should not be alone, just let me be your company,

Just the thought of you not here, it's just so strange to me,

Helpless

I do not feel like getting up, I don't feel like my normal self, Mary Jane ain't even calming me down; it seems only sleep helps,

But, it only helps because I don't have to be awake, I do not have to be aware, but even now I barely sleep, because I see you there,

I just want my peace; I need it more than anything. 'Cause the more I think of you, it becomes insanity,

I once said I did not need closure; it was the biggest lie I have ever told, the tears that I cry during meditation, remain unknown,

I wait for the message to come, your apology for what you did, but it never will, and that's some fucked up shit,

I have been crying randomly, over someone who mistreated me, as my tears fall, I just know, I am deceiving me.

Rumor Has It...

I think it is amazing how people gossip about sex. It starts off as something so innocent, but quickly develops into something everyone knows; or they think they know.

My vagina is such a blessing, that you keep speaking on it, spreading rumors just like a peasant.

Are you upset because I never sat on your face? Is this why you started this?

Honey, all you had to do was ask me, but then again you knew I was too good for you, so, it was best you didn't.

Rumor has it that I should be ashamed. But ashamed for what exactly?

Maybe you should be ashamed, that you chose to start a rumor about me; but didn't even share the good things.

You chose to try and defame what I stand for, but my grace overrides all the bullshit.

You should have shared how at 24, I am a new entrepreneur, a Black one at that.

You should have shared my cash app name, so people could know where to support my businesses.

You should have shared that I am independent, and an up and coming author.

Or maybe that I was even a funny, caring, loving person.

Instead, you chose to share something that you thought would hurt me, but you were wrong, I am not hurt.

I am just disappointed in you, because out of all rumors, this is the one you decided to choose.

Calling For Protection

Ancestors, please do not let me end up in the wrong hands again,

I don't want my sunshine and love to be ruined by another dishonest man,

I don't think there is much more I can take, not much more I can stand,

My heart does not want the pain, please do not let harm and hurt come again,

Please protect me from the evil, fake love and pretend,

Protect me from the energy, that is not of a husband,

There is not much more I can take, not much more I can stand,

Ancestors, please protect me, do not let hurt and pain come again. Ancestors, please protect me, keep me away from them.

Encouraging Friends

I remember those people who helped me through the process of being burned.

I will never forget you.

I was crying, going from burnt to bald all in one month.

How could I forget you?

Feeling ugly and trying to hide, but you all made me feel beautiful.

You said whoever called me ugly had lied, and that I was undefeatable.

With all your words of encouragement, your girl became lethal.

It was a process and I do not regret it, because my insecurities became see-through.

You helped me love myself,

Oh, how could I forget you?

You helped me love myself, I could never forget you.

Mother Earth

Today I told my mother I loved her, and for the first time in years I meant it. The amount of emotion that poured from me, almost made me tip over, because I meant it.

I have prayed for years to have real feelings, and on 5/10/2020 I think Heaven sent them.

I have grown bored of holding the past over her head, I have grown past most of my venting.

I love you mama. You are a strong woman. I can never say I went hungry.

I have been uplifting everyone except you, and that just is not right, especially since you birth me.

I cry as I write this, because I've always prayed for better.

I always wanted that bond, I wanted us to grow together.

For the first time in years, I can say this feels real.

I know I have been distant, but as they say, time heals.

I love you my Mother, my Earth, I'm glad you didn't give up.

I hope one day you open your eyes, and see that you are enough.

I cherish our time together now, you never know what can happen,

Today after I said I loved you, my heart was filled with passion.

Sisters, I Remember

I remember, oh sisters, how could I not? How could I forget our first time together, as I played Spyro on the PlayStation?

I remember we woke up that morning and ran around the room laughing. Mom was upset, so we got our ass whipped.

I remember we held each other that night because I had missed you so much.

I remember you all hid under me crying, as mom was being abused, and I told you all to hush.

I did not know how to protect you, and that itself was scary enough. I did not know if I could protect you, as we heard mommy getting beat up.

The only thing that went through my mind, is he would never harm you, as I picked the vase up. I would be on trial from protecting you, smiling with dignity, with my chin up.

As we heard the cries from mom's bedroom, I turned the tv up. I think it was raining because we were shivering, or maybe that was just us.

Our tears fell silently, because of the fear of being heard. I think you both fell asleep, but I was fully awake and still alert.

Because even though he did not hit us, our mom was still being hurt. I was so ashamed and felt so weak, because it's something she did not deserve.

Self-Worth

If you only realize your self-worth, you will realize that you are the reason the soil never dries out. Why the flowers continue to grow, and why the trees still sway high in the sky. The reason the wind blows, carrying the melodies of the birds singing joyfully and full of hope.

You are the reason why the sun blazes and shines so brightly, as if heaven has opened. You are the reason the world will continue to thrive; you are worth more than temporary love.

You are more than the anxiety that tries to overtake you. You are fearless, strong, and bold. Do not let your pain make you feel any less than a god or a goddess, no one can take your throne.

You should know and understand your self-worth, be aware of who you are. You are worth everything and more, my darling you are a god.

Imagine Being A Flower

A Sunflower in fact, because I love those, no matter the change of seasons, it will still grow,

A Sunflower which could not be used as a victim, I know my Angels are laughing at me, saying "Damn, you sure know how to pick 'em.",

Becoming deeply rooted, taking everything without asking, you'd be a fool if you tried to break me, I've been through too much to give in,

Sunflowers have become an important part of me, almost more calming than the Hen, keeping me on track, to become a better person than back then.

Black Man

You have come too far, so do not give up now,

You have come too far, so do not turn back now,

No worries, I hear your cries of despair,

No worries, even kings have moments of fear,

Do not be ashamed, I'm aware you're just a man,

I'm aware of the battles you face daily, and the hurt that is buried within,

Fake love, fake hope-- honey, where do I begin?

I know you're tired of trying to cope, so, you end up committing heavy sins,

But, darling you are still a king,

Honey, you just need a resolution,

You are still a king, Black Man,

Sometimes it just gets confusin'.

Simple Conversation

How are you? May I ask you this question?

Such a simple one it is, but it can leave such an impression,

It is amazing how words, can change a person's reflection,

You can speak love into them, or use your words to neglect them,

It does not cost anything to uplift, not one cent to love a person,

You don't sacrifice anything to give love, so why do we treat it as a burden?

Speaking positivity into someone, can be so life changin',

Speaking positive words to someone, can bring love into the equation.

Sunshine, Sunshine

We are a team, and we work as one,

Don't go too far from your body, you know what will come,

Get your crystals, purify your air, and your home,

This is a place where they're not welcome, and surely don't belong,

All the answers you need, have always been within you,

Put your faith in your Ancestors,

And watch how they'll defend you,

I'm sure it is a surprise,

That you are a Child of the Sun, and that cannot be denied,

 A Child of the Day, a protector of the light,

Your Angels have always been near, just tucked out of sight.

Mentor 101

My mentor once told me, "If they cannot handle you when you are turning into the Hulk, then they do not deserve to be in your life."

Ever since then, I have been single.

Thanks, Mentor.

I owe it all to you!

16 Positive Mantras

I Am A Goddess

I Am Greatness

I Am Loyal

I Am Free

I Am Fierce

I Am Protective

I Am Beautiful

I Am Complete

I Am Consistent

I Am Successful

I Am Intelligent

I Am Humble

I Am Unique

I Am Fearless

I Am Worthy

I Am Joyful

My happiness allows others to be happy

It's Raining Black Men

Black man, I mean, Black men. Thank you, for those who stick by our sides and hear us out.

Thank you, for those who still love us when we do not love ourselves.

Thank you, for being strong and feeding our mental health.

Thank you, for giving so much of yourself up, to make sure we are well.

I wish I could melt into your skin, and fall into your bloodstream.

That way I would always stay in your system, and you could never avoid me.

Black men you make us feel safe, created from gold and royalty.

I pray you do not give up on us, please continue to protect your Black Queens.

Although we are independent, I swear we need your love to survive.

It's just that our current circumstances, makes us question that sometimes.

And we all know too well when one is afraid, it brings unwanted pride.

But truth be told, no one really wants to be alone, for the rest of their life.

We allow our past to take a toll on what we have present, but ladies with that mindset, you just might miss your blessing.

I have been hurt back-to-back, so I understand the feeling. But how fair is it to take such anger out, on a man who is willing?

My Black men I ask you to be patient, because most of us need healing.

We are just going through phases, dealing with past trauma and demons.

Stay In Your Lane

I will do what you want, and I will do as you say, cover my scars with makeup, but the pain will remain,

We wonder why people off themselves, well, maybe because they feel drained; society's ridiculous standards will make you feel insane,

And "oh Lord", please don't level-up, because they will assume you've changed, and I'm sure you did, just not in a negative way,

Therefore, I don't mind being lonely, I try to keep my distance from the fake, I'm telling you all to protect your energy, So, it's best to just stay in your lane.

What Is Hard?

You think you have it hard, until you see the homeless people.

Until you see on tv how many innocent children are beaten and raped.

Until you see how many starving kids there really are, almost as if the numbers never end.

Until you see little kids literally taking care of themselves.

Until you see that some people never even had the chance, it was already too late.

Until you see that we are still identified as a color and not as a human being.

Until you see even after 100 years, the hate has not changed, but we can only hope for the best and try to do better.

I can only pray for the best and hope we will do better.

We should all meditate and rest, believe it will get better.

We can only manifest for the best, and just know it will get better.

To My Hood

I'm trying to have the same joyful spirit I had when I was a little girl. I remember laying on a pallet in front of my aunt's house as I fell asleep.

I didn't have to worry about being snatched, because the community was creep free. I didn't have to worry about being shot, the gangs had some type of peace.

We have gotten to that place where it is normal to say, "rest in peace." Going to a different friend's funeral, almost every day of the week.

I pray for protection over the young, I hope they see more than the streets. I know the TV portrays you as everything else, except for kings and queens.

But, honey, I ask you not to lose faith, this is just a phase, not where our people end. Ask yourself when you are angry, is it worth it, to never speak to that person again.

Do not wait 'til the day of their funeral, to apologize for something you never meant. I promise you'll regret it, and be upset with yourself for the messages you never sent.

I Ended Up In The Hospital

All I remember is waking up, and that I needed to go to work. Instead, my body would not move, I just sat weeping as I stared at the celling.

I felt like a failure, because I wasn't strong enough to get up and go to work. I am used to fixing things myself.

Panicking, thinking I would lose my job, and lose everything I had worked so hard for, because I was weak.

Calling the help line, with suicide on my mind. Wondering if I died today, would anybody even mind?

Would they come and check on me, if I didn't answer the phone?

Or would it take me not showing up to work, to realize something was wrong?

No one loves me, I think something is wrong. I am not worthy of life; it has to be why no one calls my phone.

Reaching out to my boss, I just know I let him down. This is so embarrassing, I bet he's sick of me now.

I hung my head in shame, as they directed me to help; A place where people go, involving Mental Health.

Who I Am

I Am Balanced,

I Am Mentally Wealthy,

I Am Open To Positive Changes,

I Can Manifest Anything That I Want,

I Succeed In All That I Do,

I Respect Other's Feelings, And Their Point Of View,

I Am Here To Be Guidance,

To Be A Guide On What To Do.

I Am Spiritually Ascending,

My Feelings Are Becoming Bulletproof,

I Am Elevating,

I Am Destined For Greatness Too,

No Room For Hesitation,

Just Looking For Ways To Improve.

Medication

Taking these pills, I kind of feel like an addict, although they are prescribed, I often wonder if I can manage, if I can go a full 24 hours, without thinking I have to have it,

Sometimes they help me feel calm, helping me manage the flashbacks, but they mostly keep me from flippin' on bitches, when I think I need to snap back,

My hands get to shaking, and that's when I know my anxiety's hanging by a thread, I overthink the thoughts of others, and think they are threats,

But it's all better when I take my meds,

My medication just subdues my real emotions; in the meantime, I am not actually dealing with the root cause,

This is not my cure; it is just a high to numb me from expressing my true emotions,

I know this is something mentally I must correct, but I am also aware that it takes time. In no way am I shaming anyone for needing medication. Sometimes we need that help. Never let the medication control you as if it's a necessity.

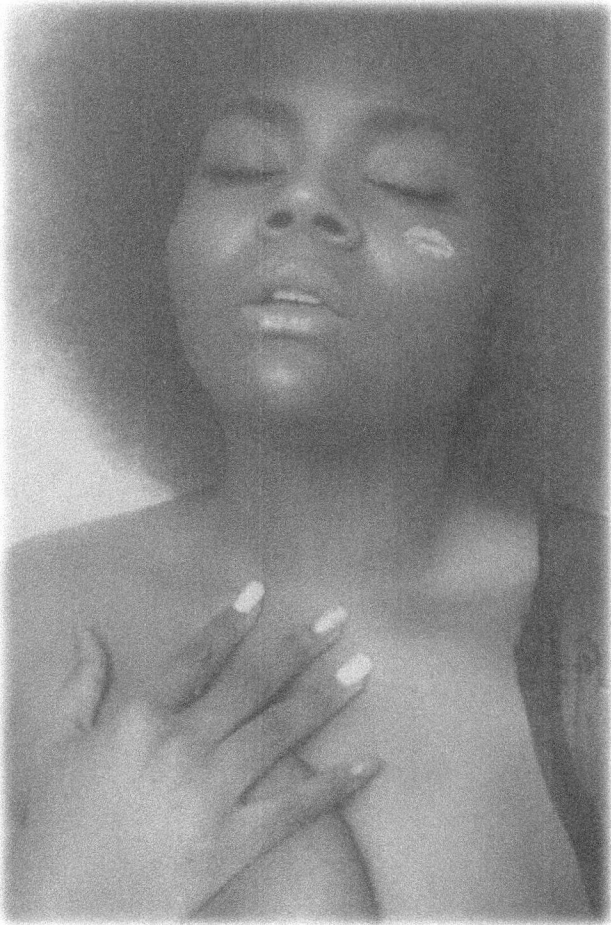

The Fire

I woke up earlier today than I normally would. I had decided to do something positive with my day. Glancing at my phone, I slid my feet to the floor as I reached for my sage.

"Today was going to be a productive day!" I thought as I fired up the sage, asking my ancestors to bless me.

Rushing into the living room with a false flash of excitement, I asked Google to play Jhene; that's my vibe, of course. Nodding my head, I began to make my morning cinnamon and ginger tea.

"I'm going to repot you, baby", I cooed to my plants.

Feeling guilty because I should have done it sooner, I was being a bad parent. Popping my ass, I danced my way into the bathroom to gather myself. Ya girl had a mission to do today, and besides I wanted to hit the stores before they got too crowded.

After gathering myself, I went to buy some soil from Home Depot. Of course, I purchased some new plants as well.

"Damn this sun is really trying a bitch!" I said, rushing back into my apartment.

"These plants better not ever die." I mumbled, as I dropped the soil on the ground.

Once on my patio, I glanced across to the buildings ahead and I saw a flicker. "I know these muhfuckas ain't barbecuing on the deck", I said in disbelief.

The flicker soon grew as the wind blew, and that's when the blood rushed from my face and went to my toes. Jumping up, I ran outside barefoot screaming "FIRE!!"

I even skipped some of the stairs in the process of trying to reach the nearest door. Banging on the first door that was in reach, I heard a man yell from behind it.

Peaking his head outside he said, "What's going on?"

I stood there for a second in shock before I spoke. My mouth tried to form a sentence, but I was frozen.

"The building is on fire!" I finally was able to get those words out, as I was breathing heavily.

Acting quickly, he turned and began yelling to his family and they ran out the door in devastation. Other neighbors soon began to gather around, running into the building trying to help in any way that they could.

"Someone is still in that apartment!" I cried out in panic.

"Oh no, what have I done?" I said to myself, walking in the direction of my car.

I was trying to make sense of things, my heart felt heavy. I felt like a failure, like I hadn't been brave enough; Why didn't I do more? I called the police as I sat in my car, explaining what was happening.

Then I dialed the one person who could help me understand. Once he answered the phone, I broke. Gasping for air, my brain was trying to find the right words to say to him.

Would he think I had failed?

How could I tell the one person that I never wanted to disappoint, that I was not brave enough to knock on *"that door?"* I was even questioning what type of person I was, because in my head if they died, it would have been my fault.

Calming me down, he tried to assure me that everything was ok, and to just wait for help. I decided I needed to walk after ending the call. I needed to feel the air against my skin, so I could stay grounded.

I flopped down in the grass, and this grey bulldog began to lick my hands. His owner sat watching the building burn down. The woman seemed distressed as she rocked back and forth in defeat.

"Which apartment is yours?" I asked, while petting the dog.

"That's our apartment on fire." she replied.

I felt a wave of relief wash over me, but the shame was still there. They could have died because I was not brave enough to knock on *"that door"*.

For Nikki

I am so lost, I cannot explain this feeling,

In fact, this just seems so unreal,

Even though I know you are somewhere in the heavens,

I would still rather have you here,

We all have our flaws,

Of course, some are worse than others.

But at the end of the day no matter what,

I will always love you, my brother,

They say you are gone,

But I refuse to accept that as truth,

Even though I feel your spirit caressing me,

Telling me to be bulletproof,

But brother I am still in shock,

Tell me why I cannot keep you?

We had plans and we have stories,

I tell you, your sister is so confused,

If I can't hear your voice again,

Wtf is the use?

If I cannot hear your voice again,

Wtf is the use?

"This is your brother speaking, Nikki, please don't lose your sight,

I know you losing me is tough, and I know you won't heal overnight,

But you're one of the bravest women I know, so I hate to see you cry,

When you think of me sister, write me letters; I promise you I'll reply,

I'll visit you when you're asleep, and tuck you in at night,

Kissing your tears as they fall from your face, giving you strength to fight,

When you think of me, look at the children, baby sister please continue to fight!

Be strong and think of me, I promise I'll visit you tonight."

Message From The Author

I often wonder what the hell love is....

Is it good or bad, or is it more than heartbreak?

Well, I must tell you, I finally experienced love in 2020. It was the most difficult love at first, but what I got in the end was so worth it.

"What love is this?" you may ask.

It is Self-Love.

We control what we attract, and we can control our emotions. Although it can be time consuming, and scary, you will find yourself smiling at the end of the process.

I sat in my bed for almost four months feeling empty. I had forgotten who I was, and where I belonged.

Then one day I woke up, and I wanted to challenge myself. I started to set boundaries, determined to become the change I wanted to be.

Try not to just lie in the pain, or your disappointments. Then again, are disappointments really disappointments, or is that just another way to challenge yourself?

This process made me open parts of my soul, that I truly wished to hide. I had to learn to love myself, even the self that made mistakes and said hurtful things.

Reflecting on myself was the most painful part of this process because I didn't know who I was. It seemed like everyone else had an idea except for me, and that was one of the most frightening things of all.

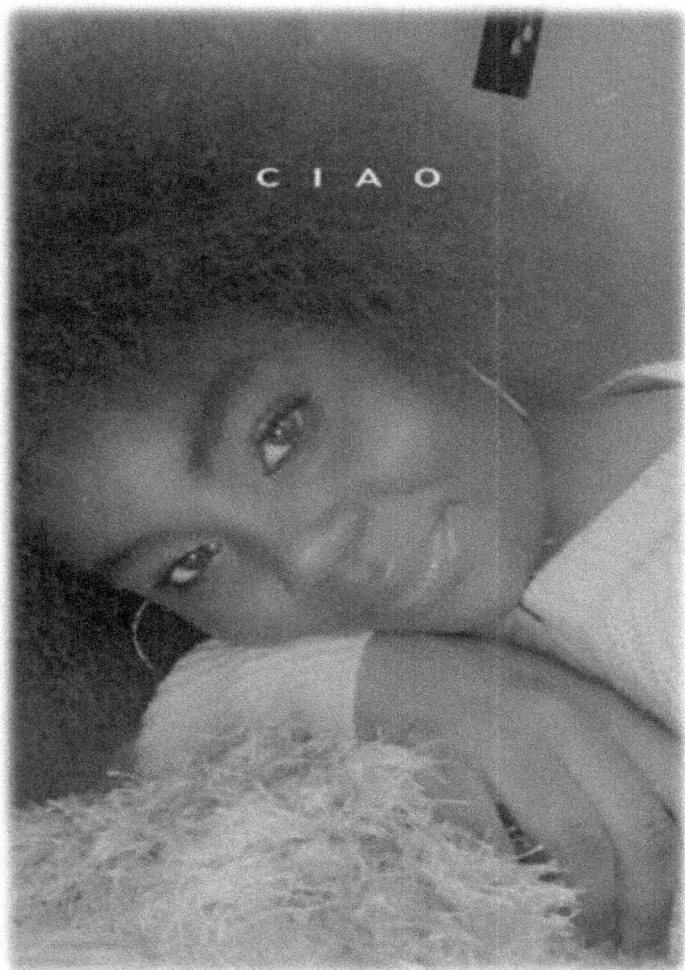

CIAO

Rambling (Song)

I am truly divine, full of love and joy.
Laying in the sun, refueling my spirit.
Before I go to war, with anyone or anything that tries to
hold me back.

I have been going to therapy,
Hoping they could help fix me.
My wounds have not healed just yet,
Still today it affects me.

I have problems with abandonment,
Saying baby please, do not leave me.
But I still get up and smile,
I refuse to let life break me.

Never going down without a fight,
It just would not be right.

Oh, it is so hard,
To get up and look beyond the stars.
Oh, it is so hard to get up and not cry.
I have been tossing and turning, every fucking night.
Not knowing, if I want to live or die.

I have been blessed,
To have a couple of friends.
Trying not to stress,
On what is not and focus on what is.

Taking my medication,
That tells me how to feel.
It makes me so damn calm,

I forget that I am real.

I have problems with abandonment,
Saying baby please, do not leave me.
But I still get up and smile,
I refuse to let life break me.

Never going down without a fight,
It just would not be right.

Oh, it is so hard,
To get up and look beyond the stars.
Oh, it is so to get up and not cry.
I have been tossing and turning, every fucking night.
Not knowing, if I want to live or die.

Choices...

Standards?

It had been a while since I let someone dig deep in my guts, in fact it had been 6 months. So, I know my pussy was tighter than the cap on a glass Coca Cola Bottle.

"Maybe I want some dick." I thought.

"Beep, Beep!" The cars behind me blew their horns.

"Shit!" I breathed, forgetting I was even driving.

Folks, always be aware of your surroundings. Here I am in traffic, thinking about dick. I pulled into the lot of my favorite gas station, I needed to grab some things.

"How are you?" The cashier asked me.

"I'm doing good, it was a long day at work today."

"Where do you work again?"

"Marshals distribution center." I replied, handing him my money.

"I'll see you later man." Winking, I walked out the door.

As I began to pump my gas, I heard a voice from behind. Turning around I saw this dude, who had two crunched up braids, going to the back of his head. Instantly I was turned off, and wondered what did this nigga want?

"Hey, what's up?" I questioned him.

"I saw some things that you bought in there, and I got some dro from Cali." He replied.

"Shit why not." I thought. But I knew one thing, he looked like he had drunk too much beer. Nothing wrong with a chunky nigga, shit, I'm chunky; but it is something about how he carried himself that I was not fucking with.

"Yeah, I'll take some."

"Aight"

He rushed back to his car to do his thing, as I waited in mine, ready to go. He opened the door and slid in, handing me my package in the process. From eyeing it I could tell he was on bullshit.

"You short."

He looked at me,

"I can show you it's not."

"Then show me, because you short." I responded.

Opening the door, he went back to his car. Long story short, the nigga was short. And yeah, he had to run me mines; I just wanted what I paid for. We exchanged numbers, and that's when shit went left. The nigga started texting for shit other than what I needed, he wanted the pussy.

Now I know what y'all thinkin', because frankly I was thinkin' it too. But ya girl pussy was in heat, and although I wasn't into it, I wanted to play. I entertained it for about two weeks, then invited him over.

"America!" This was the oddest shit ever, mainly because I did not really want to do the shit; so why was I about to go through with this shit?

Going into my room he bent me over, as he pulled his pants down. But it was something about the way his stomach was smacking against my ass, I did not like. He would get his nut, but I was shit out of luck.

But in that moment, I realized something. I realized that in those six months, I had outgrown a lot of my old habits. Shit like this just was not entertaining anymore, and I was ok with being alone.

After he nutted, I was more wishing he would just leave. He tried to have a conversation, I replied with a yawn; picking up my signal he headed towards the door.

"So, alright", he said, or something like that as he walked out the door.

"Drive safe." I said, closing the door.

"I'm so over this lame shit." I huffed as I headed to the shower.

The lesson here is, ladies never lower your standards, remember your worth and who you are.

Nobody's Victim

Listen up people, stay the fuck back!
I'm the realness that you say you want, but when you get
it, you don't know how to act,

I'm loyal to all my bitches, and there is no lie in that,
Don't listen to da gossip, that shit'll get you smacked,

Got no energy for weak minded individuals, and that's
no cap,
Don't pull no gun, if you ain't gone shoot it, with your
bubble head ass,

Boy you not hot, you're a loser, face mask smelling like
ass,
And bitch you're a groupie, you're an option, with your
dick sucking ass,

You think I'm weak? Nah, I just move with class,
I try to walk away from drama, to prevent me, from
losing everything that I have,

A lot of you hoes wanna see me lose, but that's just too
bad,
'Cause anything the divine has given me, ain't up for
grabs,

With that being said, I'm nobody's victim, I can, and will
beat your ass,
Whether it's these hands, or this mouth, speaking
common knowledge, you've never had,

You think you're a threat, lol, neva dat,
I'll take everything you got, while being legal, in the
process,

It be dem victims, that ain't scared to move, when it's
time to act,
It be dem victims that y'all call scary, that would put a
nigga in bags,

Keeping all of your secrets, like how you out here eating
ass,
Banging your homeboy's wife, while he doin' time for
your crime, that shit super sad,

I'm only a victim to the system, with they white ass,
But even they got me fucked up, 'cause I fight back,

I'm too royal, too lovely, to accept anything less,
And if you can't see that, then this is where we split, no
communication left,

I ain't nobody's victim, so step the fuck back.

Vivid Dreams

Oh, a bitch was loyal and dumb,

Refusing to see the red flags, because the nigga was handsome,

Having vivid dreams, about him killing the pussy, before I even met em,

Imagining sucking him off, practicing, with a grapefruit and banana,

I wasn't givin da pussy away to no other nigga, keeping it tight building up stamina,

Bitin' my pillow, as I played with my pussy, imagining I was riding him,

Havin that dick brick hard, while my pussy juices surrounded 'em,

Pinching my titties, I licked my lips, this pussy would earn some miles from him,

If he's anything, like I imagine, I might just say fuck it, and have a child by 'em,

Getting closer to my orgasm, I opened my legs wide, so I could cum for him,

I heard a knock, on my door, "fuck!", I was interrupted; I guess I would miss my nut again.

Misunderstood

You will never truly know me, I have a hard time trying to find myself,

Hard on the outside, but within I'm softer than cotton,

There are too many layers to me, I've lost track when countin',

People are attracted to me, because I'm something mysterious,

Tryin' to have unnecessary conversations, because they are curious,

They get with me, thinking they could handle this,

Instead, they runaway, when it gets tough, abort mission, abandonment,

I am misunderstood, on many different levels, and when people don't understand, they tend to give you a label,

If I don't speak enough, then I'm deemed as rude, or not mentally capable,

If I speak too loud, then I'm reckless, childish, and unstable,

Just because we have a conversation, don't think that you know me,

Depending on the day and mood, I have different personalities,

The walls that I have built, protects me from unholy enemies,

It takes time and endurance, to even understand a fraction of me,

I let people form their own opinions, of what they think of me,

They don't know the half, only what I show em, I can be who you want me to be,

My soul is very versatile, have fun tryin' to get a hold of me,

One minute I'm open, then I'm closed off, it'll take a lifetime to understand me.

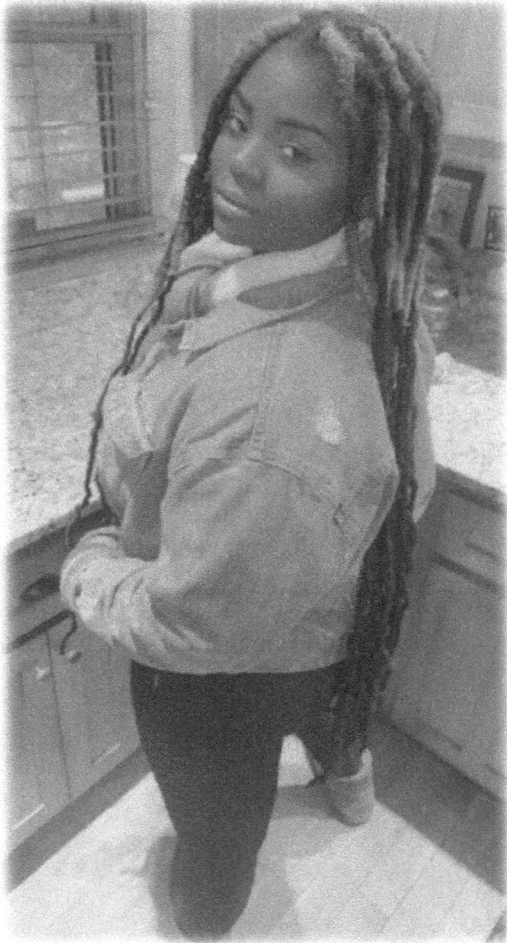

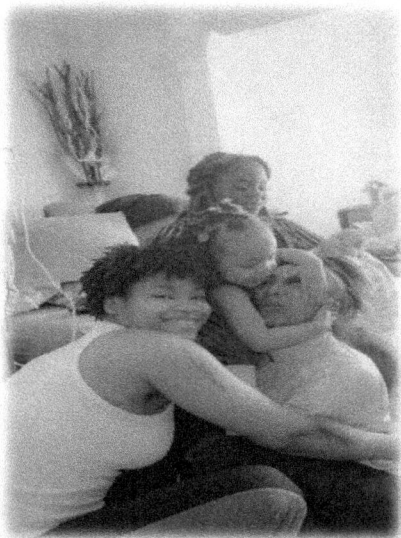

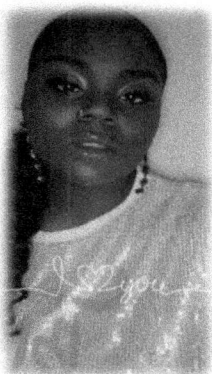

Fat, My First + Second Niece, Rre

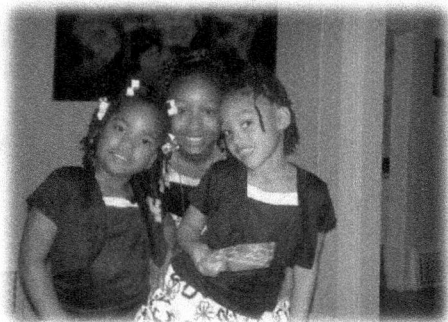

TaeTae, Rre, Twinky

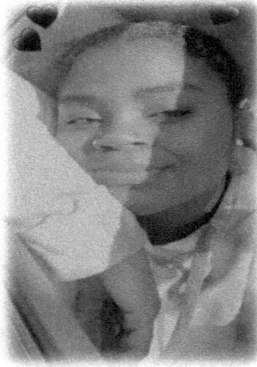

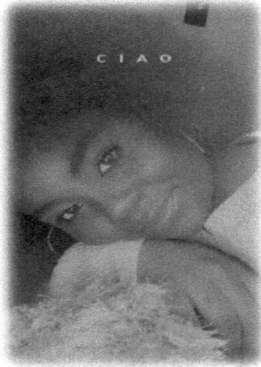

My Sexy Ass

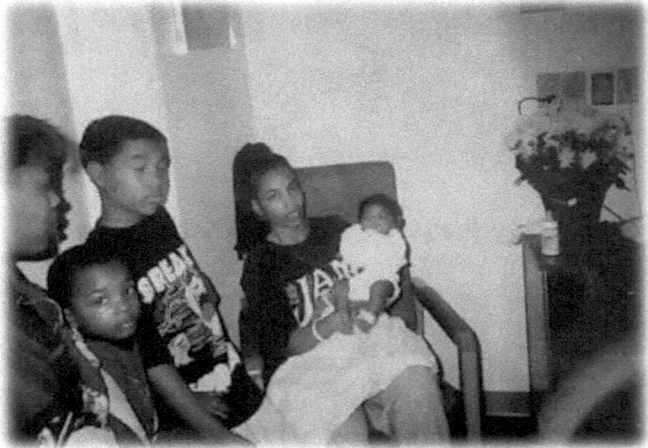

My Grandmother, Uncle Jerome, Uncle Harold

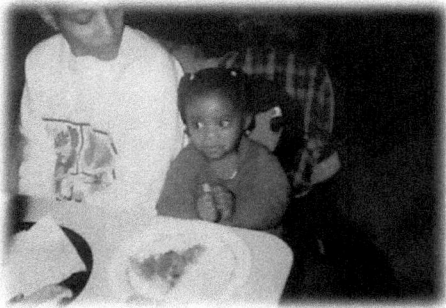

My Grandmother and I

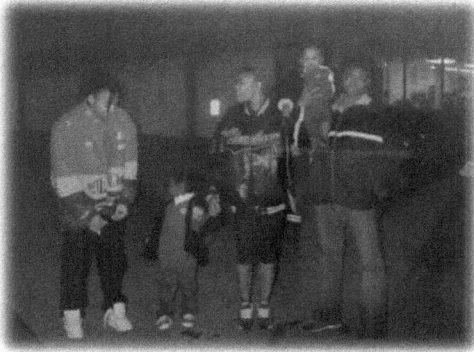

Aunt Shakeeta, Aunt Sharonda, My
Aunt Shara, Me in the blue

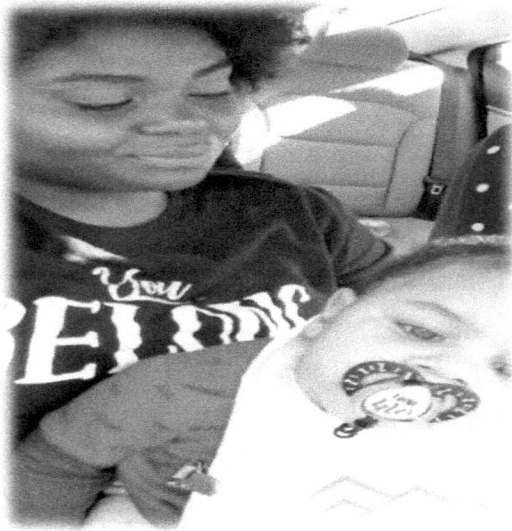

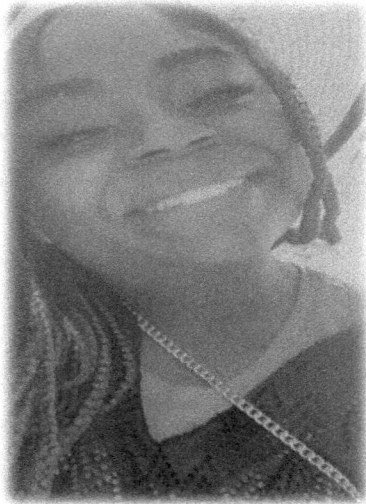

King and I

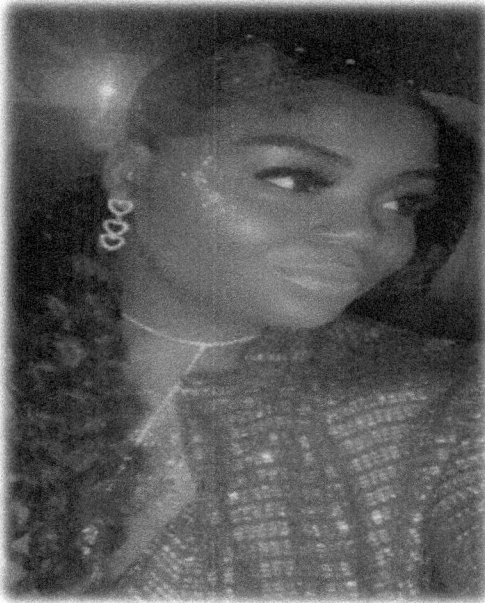

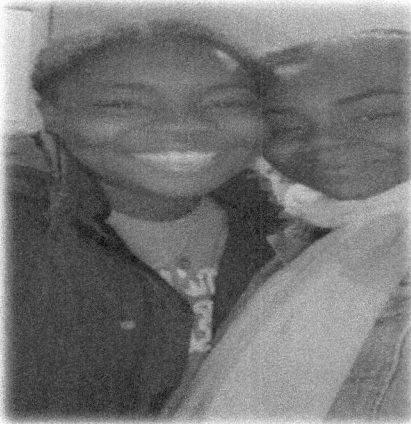

One of my close friends, Christian

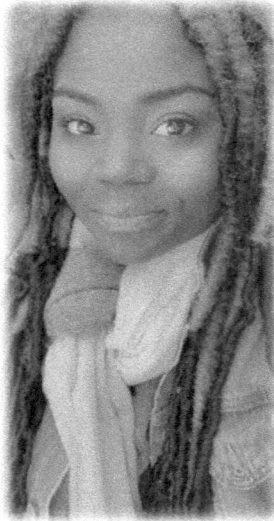

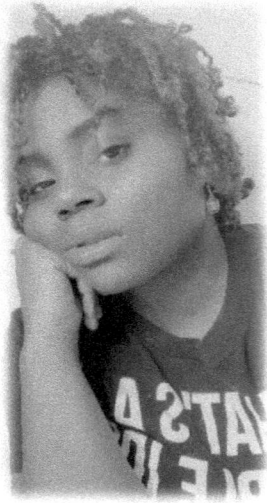

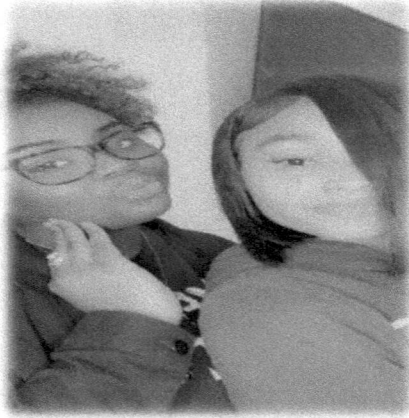

My sister Twinky

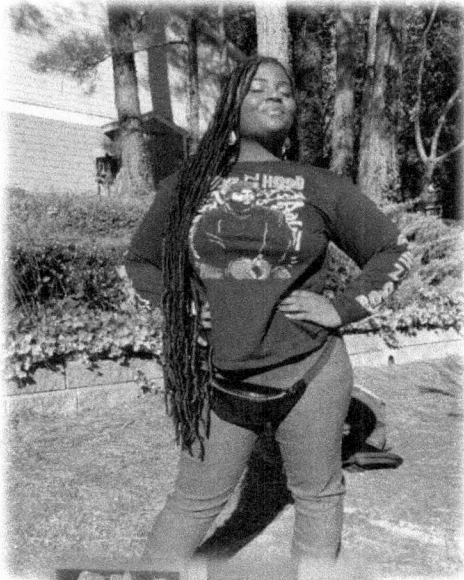

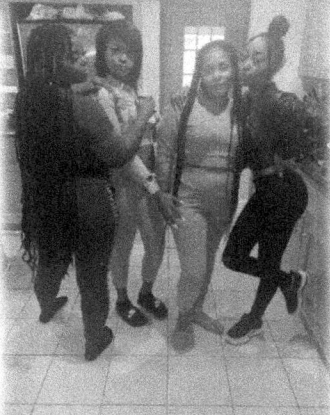

My Sister's, and Mother

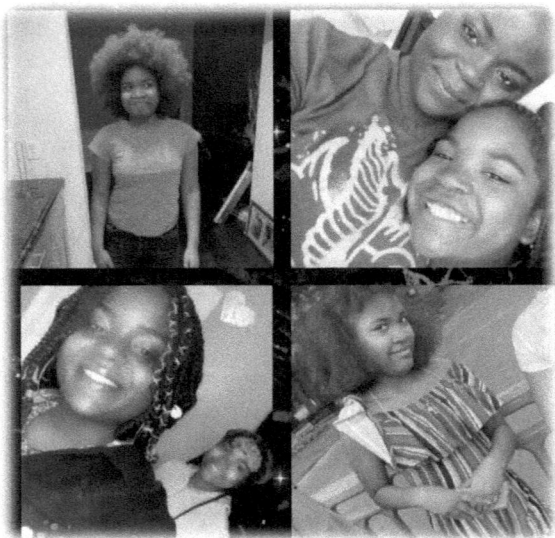

My Sister TaeTae and I

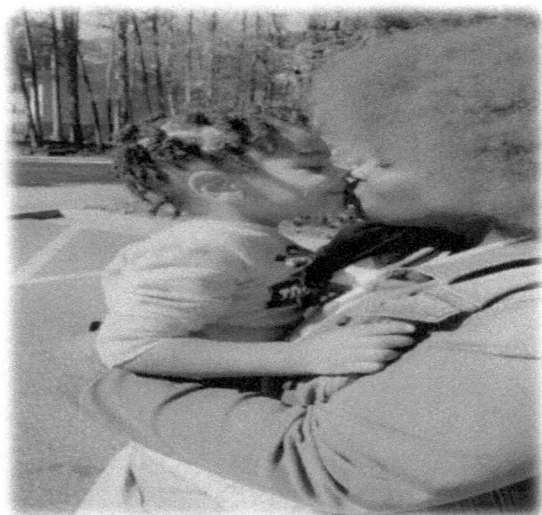

King

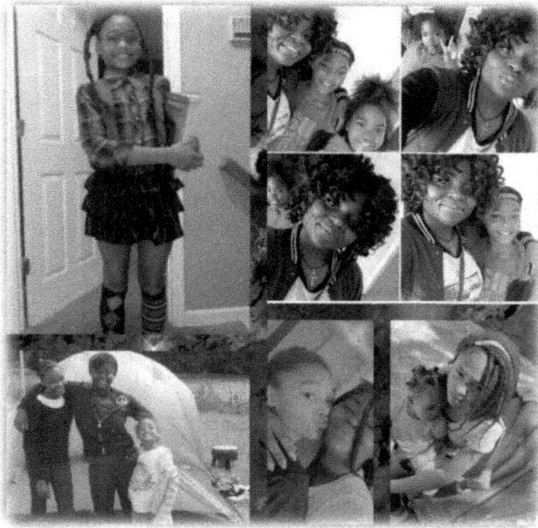

My Sister Twinky

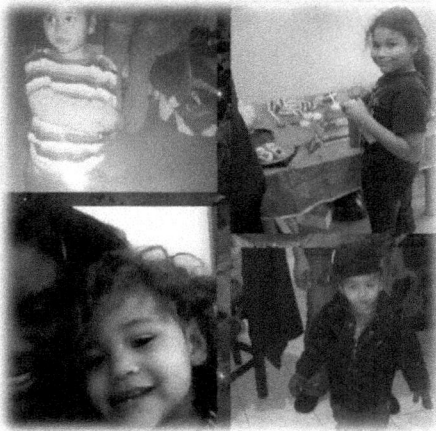

My one and only Brother

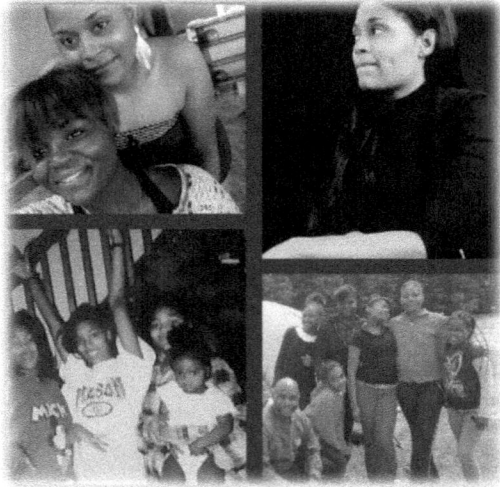

My Mother

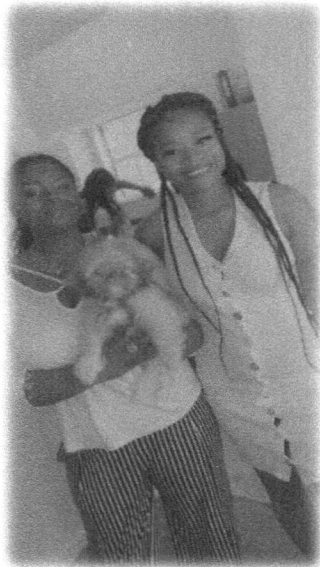

My Sister Fat

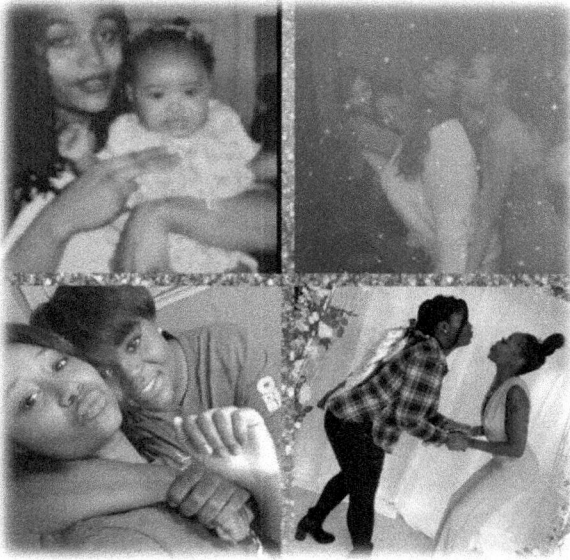

My Sister Rre and I

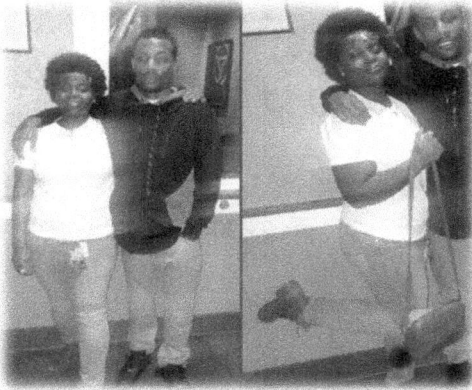

My Uncle Shamar

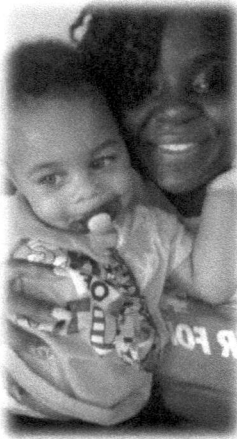
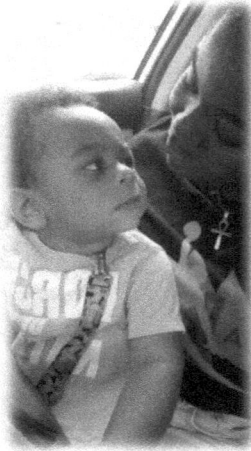

King and I

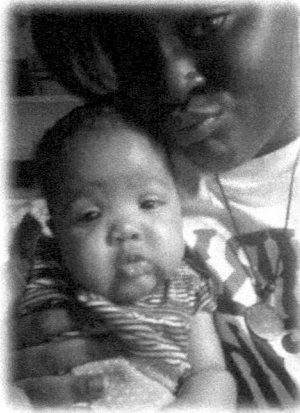
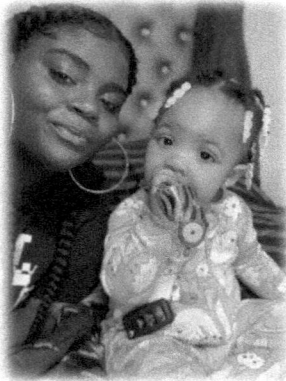

My 1ˢᵗ Niece

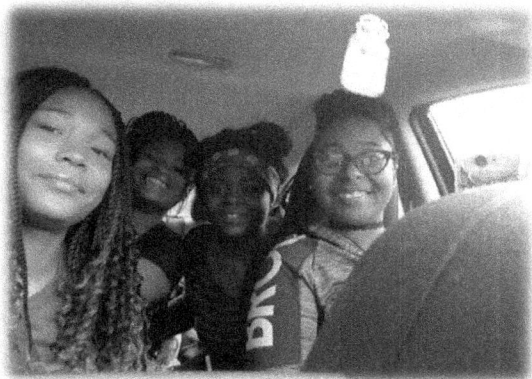

Aunt Sharice, My Sister Fat, My Sister Breonna

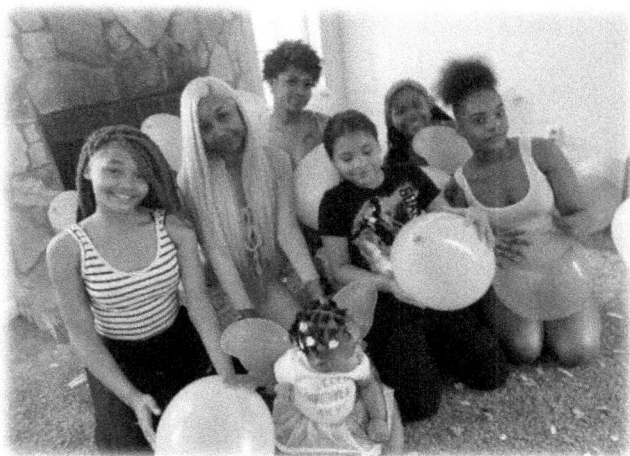

All my sibling's, and my first Niece.

I love you,
I love you,
I see you,
And I love you,

www.ingramcontent.com/pod-product-compliance
Lightning Source LLC
Chambersburg PA
CBHW060515280326
41933CB00014B/2979